Asmaa Kadhim Al-Sarraji
Rajaa Al-Tikreeti

Misoprostol in Midtrimester Termination of Pregnancy

Asmaa Kadhim Al-Sarraji
Rajaa Al-Tikreeti

Misoprostol in Midtrimester Termination of Pregnancy

Oral and Vaginal Misoprostol in Midtrimester Termination of Pregnancy

LAP LAMBERT Academic Publishing

Impressum / Imprint
Bibliografische Information der Deutschen Nationalbibliothek: Die Deutsche Nationalbibliothek verzeichnet diese Publikation in der Deutschen Nationalbibliografie; detaillierte bibliografische Daten sind im Internet über http://dnb.d-nb.de abrufbar.
Alle in diesem Buch genannten Marken und Produktnamen unterliegen warenzeichen-, marken- oder patentrechtlichem Schutz bzw. sind Warenzeichen oder eingetragene Warenzeichen der jeweiligen Inhaber. Die Wiedergabe von Marken, Produktnamen, Gebrauchsnamen, Handelsnamen, Warenbezeichnungen u.s.w. in diesem Werk berechtigt auch ohne besondere Kennzeichnung nicht zu der Annahme, dass solche Namen im Sinne der Warenzeichen- und Markenschutzgesetzgebung als frei zu betrachten wären und daher von jedermann benutzt werden dürften.

Bibliographic information published by the Deutsche Nationalbibliothek: The Deutsche Nationalbibliothek lists this publication in the Deutsche Nationalbibliografie; detailed bibliographic data are available in the Internet at http://dnb.d-nb.de.
Any brand names and product names mentioned in this book are subject to trademark, brand or patent protection and are trademarks or registered trademarks of their respective holders. The use of brand names, product names, common names, trade names, product descriptions etc. even without a particular marking in this works is in no way to be construed to mean that such names may be regarded as unrestricted in respect of trademark and brand protection legislation and could thus be used by anyone.

Coverbild / Cover image: www.ingimage.com

Verlag / Publisher:
LAP LAMBERT Academic Publishing
ist ein Imprint der / is a trademark of
AV Akademikerverlag GmbH & Co. KG
Heinrich-Böcking-Str. 6-8, 66121 Saarbrücken, Deutschland / Germany
Email: info@lap-publishing.com

Herstellung: siehe letzte Seite /
Printed at: see last page
ISBN: 978-3-659-43691-8

Copyright © 2013 AV Akademikerverlag GmbH & Co. KG
Alle Rechte vorbehalten. / All rights reserved. Saarbrücken 2013

Misoprostol in Midtrimester Termination of Pregnancy

Asmaa K. Al-Sarraji
(M.B.CH.B.,F.I.B.O.G,C.A.B.O.G.)
College of Medicine
Babylon University
IRAQ

Rajaa A. Al-Tikreeti
MRCOG
College of Medicine
Baghdad University
IRAQ

List of contents

	page
Introduction	3
Termination of pregnancy	3
Indications of termination of pregnancy	3
Methods of termination	4
Surgical methods	5
Complications of pregnancy termination	6
Medical methods	7
Prostaglandins and termination of pregnancy	10
Natural PGs	10
Synthetic PGs	11
Misoprostol	12
Chemical structure of misoprostol	12
Mechanism of action of misoprostol	14
Pharmacokinetics of misoprostol	14
Side effects of misoprostol	15
Over dose and toxicity	17
Contraindications and warnings	17
Indications and usages of misoprostol	18
Advantages of misoprostol	19
Teratogenisity of misoprostol	19
Routes of administrations	20
Dosage and dosing interval	21
Aim of the study	24
Materials and methods	25
Results	29
Discussion	43
Conclusions	51
Recommendations	52
References	53

INTRODUCTION

Termination of pregnancy:

Termination of pregnancy is removal or ending of pregnancy without any expectation that the fetus will survive. The gestational limit is determined by legal status in each country and varies considerably. In some countries it is possible to terminate pregnancy at any gestation [1].

Although abortion related mortality and morbidity increase significantly as gestation advanced, induction of abortion after 14 weeks of gestation is associated with sharp rise in the rate of complication and in consequent medical cost.[2]

Indication of termination of pregnancy

1. Fetal indication:

Prenatal diagnosis has progressed, but most condition diagnosed has no real means of treatment other than abortion. Fetal indication for induced abortion include those anatomic condition incompatible with life (e.g. anencephaly) and major congenital abnormalities (e.g. hypoplastic Lt heart) .When the condition is diagnosed in the time to have an abortion 50-80 % of patient selected abortion.[3]

Other fetal indication for TOP is intrauterine fetal death which is a common problem in obstetric practice. This condition may be complicated by psychological problems, infection, and consumptive coagulopathy .For physician confronted with IUD the management of this condition posses a dilemma, although a significant number of of these patients go in labor within several weeks ,others do not.[4]

2. Maternal indication:

Medical indications for abortion have narrowed with advances in perinatal care. In 1980s it was estimated that maternal mortality was reduced seven folds by 1st trimester abortion.

Maternal conditions that may be considered under medical indication include:

- Renal failure
- Diabetic retinopathy
- Neoplasia
- Psychiatric disorders
- Cardiac conditions that may result in maternal mortality include severe mitral stenosis, coaractation of aorta and uncorrected tetralogy of Fallot.

A cardiac condition with potentially greater mortality is Eisenmenger syndrome with pulmonary hypertension. [3]

Methods of TOP

The objective of any method of pregnancy termination are to provide safe acceptable technique for both patient and saff,cause the lowest risk possible for future health, fertility and pregnancy outcome.[1]

These methods either surgical or medical

1. Surgical methods

Surgical termination of pregnancy present increasing hazard proportionate to the gestational age, this is because the fetal parts are bigger and the risk of tearing the cervix or damaging the uterus is greater.[5] In the 1st trimester the most widely used method is vacume aspiration or suction curettage which is used until the end of the 1st trimester.[6]

In the 2nd trimester it has been reported to be associated with 3-5 times higher morbidity and mortality risk than termination in the 1st trimester, moreover there is considerable controversy about which method is safest, produce least number of complications, the least amount of stress for the patient and is most cost effective [7]

Surgical methods include:

A. Dilatation and curettage.

This method is widely used in USA and may be performed as a day case under local anesthesia with cervical block or under general anesthesia [1].

B. Catheter and balloon

A technique used for midtrimester abortion before it was replaced by extra-amniotic PG administration. Once adequate dilatation has been achieved the catheter will pass through the cervix and balloon will present in the vagina, thereafter induction can be advanced either by low amniotomy or administration of an oxytocic [1].

C. Hysterotomy

This usually performed under general anesthesia, the care that required and complications are similar to that of women delivered of alive birth by caesarean section [1].

D. Other methods

As hygroscopic and mechanical dilators, when compared with their frequent use in the process of producing a 1st or early 2nd trimester abortion, cervical dilators have been employed with relative infrequency for the induction of labor. Hygroscopic dilators work by absorbing water by osmosis, with resulting change in their size and shape, when placed into the cervical canal over a period of hours (> 12 hrs often overnight) they produce mechanical dilatation which then permit an amniotomy to be performed, these agents also stimulate the local release of PGs which may have additional benefit on the cervical ripening [8].

Complications of pregnancy termination

The incidence of complication occurring after pregnancy termination is low, although it tends to increase with advancing gestation, to some extent the complication are related to the method of termination used with some being more common after certain procedure.

These complications are:

1. Incomplete abortion

Incomplete abortion following medically induced late abortion is influenced by gestational age with 60% being incomplete at 12 weeks and 20% at 19 weeks gestation [1].

2. Excessive hemorrhage

The rate of uterine hemorrhage (more than 500 ml) is low, less than 5% of cases and the need for blood transfusion are exceedingly rare. Uterine atony can be decreased by complete evacuation of the uterus [3].

3. Cervical damage

Cervical laceration may occur with all methods of termination; post abortion per vaginum examination should perform to exclude this rare complication and appropriate repair surgery organized when indicated [1].

4. Endometrial adhesion

Asherman syndrome should be suspected in patient with no menses for several cycles following TOP by curettage, this is rare complication and may be avoided through the prevention of endometritis and the avoidance of post evacuation sharp curettage [3].

5. Uterine body damage

Perforation may occur with surgical approach and rupture of the body of the uterus with medical termination, damage is more common with dilatation and evacuation occurring in 0.2-1 % [1].

6. Coagulopathy

This is provoked with the use of hypertonic solutions, but not the PGs alone [1].

7. Infection

This may occur with both surgical and medical methods of managing abortion. It is more common if there is a long induction to abortion interval with medically induced abortion [1].

2. Medical methods

Medical abortion becomes the 1st choice for 2nd trimester termination of pregnancy in many countries although dilatation and evacuation is commonly used in USA [2].

Drugs used for TOP are:

A. Oxytocin

Among different dugs used for medical abortion, oxytocin has been used infrequently before 24 weeks gestation because of perceived lack of efficacy. It is not recommended in cases of fetal death with unfavorable cervix [7].

B. Mifepristone

It is proven to be used for medical abortion, initially approved in France in 1988 [9]. It is progesterone antagonist also known as RU 486 which bind to progesterone receptor with affinity 5 times as great as that of progesterone, unlike progesterone this complex inhibit transcription resulting in down regulation of progesterone-dependent gene with decidual necrosis and detachment of product of conception. It is also act on endometrial blood vessels causing damage that further compromises the embryo, these agents directly promote uterine contraction by increasing myometerial cell excitability and they also cause cervical dilatation [10].

This drug is expensive and should not be given to patients on corticosteroid therapy or who had suspected adrenal insufficiency because it binds to the glucocorticoid receptor and block the action of cortisol [11].

One of the published regimen for mid-trimester medical abortion include 200 mg oral mifepriston followed 36-48 hrs later by misoprostol 800 mcg vaginally, then review after six hrs if not progressed repeat the dose of misoprostol 800 mcg vaginally [11].

C. Methotroxate

It was also employed in early 1990s for medical termination of pregnancy [9], it is a folic acid antagonist interfere with DNA synthesis, actively proliferating cells including those from malignant tumor, bone marrow, trophoblast are sensitive to Methotroxate, so its mechanism of action is through inhibition of trophoblast development [10]. Methotroxate and Misoprostol used in combination are very effective in terminating pregnancy. Methotroxate is usually given in a dose of 50 mg per square meter of body surface area, administered by intramuscular injection, high dose (60 mg/m^2) does not increase the success rate[10]. Oral administration (25 or 50 mg) is also effective, three-seven days after the Methotroxate has been administered, and misoprostol (800 mcg) is administered by vaginal route [10].

Methotroxate had several side effects which include: skin rash, GIT ulceration, leukocyte depression, and depression of erythropoieses, alopecia, hepatocellular damage, jaundice and skin photosensitivity [12].

D. Prostoglandins (PGs)

PGs together with (thromboxanes and leukotriens) known as Eicosanoid which is the name given to a group of 20 carbon unsaturated fatty acid derived principally from Arachidonic acid in the cell wall, they are short lived, extremely potent and formed in almost every tissue in the body, their biosynthesis pathways are shown in figure (1)[13].

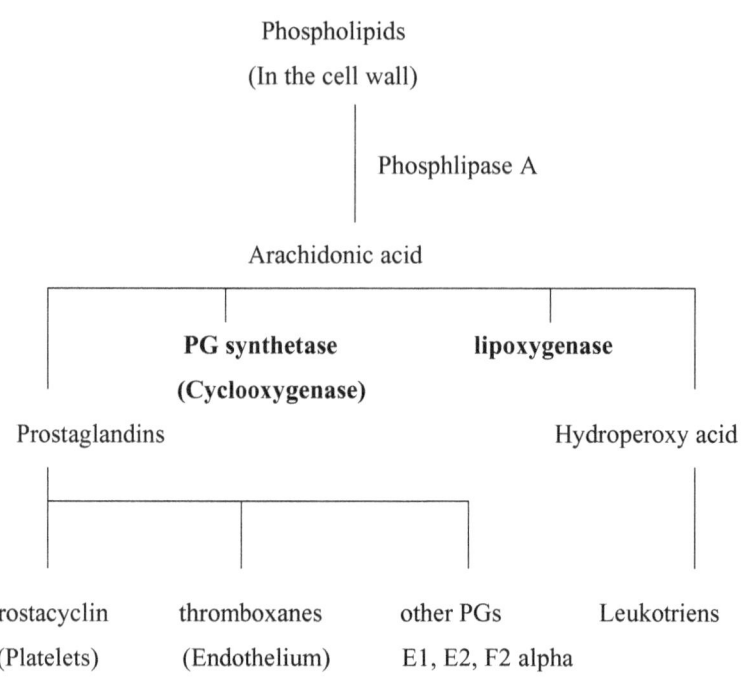

Figure(1): Biosynthetic pathway of Eicosanoid[13]

Prostaglandin and termination of pregnancy

PGs are the most common agents used to terminate the pregnancy in the second trimester either alone or after pretreatment with Mifepriston[14].

PGs either natural or synthetic

Natural PGs

It has been reported that intravenous infusion of either PG E2 or PG F2 alpha could effectively induce second trimester TOP.

Intravenous administration of effective doses of naturally occurring PG however was associated with high incidence of gastrointestinal side effect charactistically nausea, vomiting and diarrhea, further more local irritation at the infusion site was observed in up to 60% of patient, and these side effects severely curtailed the clinical utility of intravenous administration.

Intra-amniotic and intrauterine instillation was subsequently found to be effective for second trimester abortion, however this regimen required either multiple administration or continuous infusion of PG through indwelling catheter, the potential risk of infection limited the general acceptance of the technique[2].

Naturally occurring PG E1 is ineffective after oral administration because it is unstable in an acid environment[15], therefore the inherent characteristic of natural PGs i.e. rapid inactivation necessating continuous or at least frequent administration and the high incidence of gastrointestinal side effects, precluded the wide spread acceptance of these agents for TOP[2].

Synthetic PGs(analogue)

The rapid inactivation of the natural PGs, due to dehydration at carbon-15, resulted in PG metabolites that possessed greatly reduced biological activity[2]. Bundy and co-workers synthesized PG analogue which are modified at carbon-15 and resisted enzymatic degradation[16]. Synthetic PG analogues are relatively resistant to metabolism hence have prolonged action[2].

PG E and F analogue have been used for 2nd trimester abortion. The PG E analogue is preferable as it has more selective action on the myomrtrium and causes fewer gastrointestinal side effects[2].

The three most extensively studied PGs E are Sulprostone, Gemeprost and Misoprostol [2].

Sulprostone
It is PG E2 analogue was studied in the early 1980s for 2nd trimester abortion, usually given intramuscularly at adoseof 0.5 mg every four hours. Also can be used intra or extra amniotically [2].

The use of parantral analogue has been discontinued because it was associated with cardiovascular complication such as acute myocardial infarction and severe hypotension [10].

Gemeprost
Is PG E1 analogue and it is the only licensed in UK for induction of abortion. Studies using a vaginal Gemoprost only regimen gave a complete abortion rate of 88-96.5 % in 48 hours [2].

The most common regimen is 1 mg vaginally every 3 hours for five courses. The mean induction to abortion interval ranges from 14-18 hours. This drug is expensive and need to be stored in refrigerator [2].

Misoprostol
Is a synthetic analogue of naturally occurring PG E1. It has been approved by the food and drug administration to be taken orally for prevention of and treatment of gastric ulcer associated with the use of NSAIDs.() It has also become an important drug in obstetric and gynecologic practice because of its uterogenic and cervical ripening effect [17].

Chemical structure of Misoprostol
Misoprostol is synthetic (15 deoxy-16 hydroxy-16 methyl) analogue of naturally occurring PG E1 [2]. It differs structurally from PG E1 by the presence of methyl ester at carbon-1 , a methyl group at carbon-16 and hydroxyl group at carbon-16 rather than at carbon-15 [18]. It appears that a

methyl ester at carbon-1 increase the anti-secretory potency and duration of action of misoprostol while movement of hydroxy group from carbon-15 to carbon-16 and addition of a methyl group at carbon-16 improve oral activity, increase the duration of action and improve safety profile of the drug compared with those of PG E1[18,19,20].

The chemical structure of misoprostol is shown below[21]

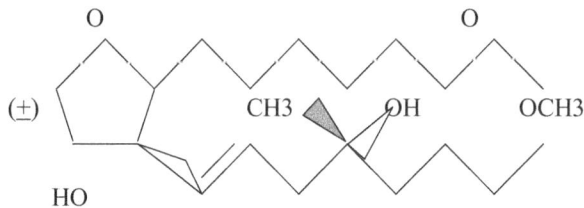

And

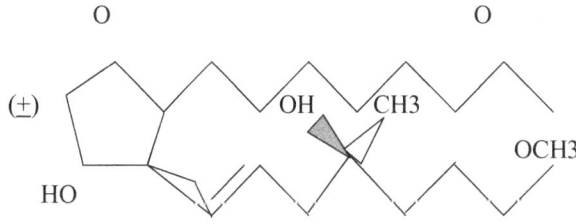

C22H38O5

± Methyl 11 (alpha 1, 16-dihydroxy-16-methyl-9 oxoprost. M.W(382.5)

Mechanism of action

1. On gastrointestinal tract

Like endogenous PG E1(cytotec) exerts a protective effect on gastrointestinal mucosa by increasing mucus and bicarbonate ion secretion and by increasing mucosal blood flow, in addition it inhibit acid secretion[21].

2. On Reproductive tract

Like other PGs it induces cervical ripening which is a complex process that involves in the physical softening and distensibility of the cervix.

The process involve action of enzymatic dissolution of collagen fibrils within the cervix, an increase in water content of the cervix and chemical changes that contribute to the clinical finding of cervical effacement and early dilatation[22]. So PGs induced ripening is associated with enzymatic collagen degradation and increase water content in the cervical extra cellular matrix[23]. Independent of their local effect on the cervix, PG also stimulates the myometrium resulting in uterine contraction and possibly hyperstimulation[23].

Pharmacokinetic of misoprostol

Absorption

Misoprostol is manufactured as an oral preparation after oral administration it is rapidly absorbed from gastrointestinal tract and converted to its pharmacologically active metabolite-misoprostol acid- plasma concentration of which peaks in approximately 30 minutes and decline thereafter[17].

Food and anti acid decease the rate of absorption of misoprostol resulting in delayed and decrease peak plasma concentration of misoprostol acid[24,25]

Metabolism

Misoprostol is primarily metabolized in the liver[17] and undergoes extensive and rapid first pass metabolism (de-esterfication) to form misoprostol acid (free acid) ,the principle and active metabolite of the drug[18,24].

Excretion

Following oral administration of misoprostol , the free acid and other metabolites of the drug are excreted mainly in the urine[24,26], smaller amounts of metabolites are excreted in the feces probably via biliary elimination[18,26]. Only negligible amounts of unchanged drug are excreted in the urine following oral or intravenous administration[26].

Drug interactions

Misoprostol has no known drug interaction and does not induce Cytochrome P450 enzyme system[17]. There was no evidence of interaction between cytotec and cardiac , gastrointestinal ,pulmonary or central nervous system drugs[24]. Decrease bioavailability of misoprostol acid was observed with high dose of antacids[20,24].

Side effects

The side effects associated with misoprostol vary according to the dosage[27] , and are include:

1. Gastrointestinal :

Diarrhea, abdominal pain, nausea, vomiting, dyspepsia and constipation. Diarrhea was dose related and usually developed early in the course of therapy , usually was self limiting. The incidence of diarrhea can be minimized by administering the drug after meals and at bed time, and by avoiding co administration of cytotec with magnesium containing anti acids[24,28].

2. Gynecological:

Spotting, cramps, hypermenorrhea, menstrual disorder, dysmenorrhea and post menopausal vaginal bleeding[24,28].

3. Elderly:

No significant difference in the safety profile of cytotec in older compared with younger patients[21]

4. Causal relationship unknown:

The following adverse events were infrequently reported. Causal relationship between cytotec and these events have not been established but cannot be excluded[21], these include:

A. Special senses: abnormal taste, abnormal vision, earache, conjunctivitis, deafness and tinnitus[24].

B. Body as a whole: Aches, pain, asthenia, fatigue, fever, rigor and weight changes[21,24].

C. Respiratory: upper respiratory tract infection, bronchitis, bronchspasm, dyspnea and epistaxis[24].

D. Cardiovascular: chest pain, edema, hypotension, hypertension, arrhythmia, phlebitis, increase cardiac enzymes and syncope[21,24].

E. Gastrointestinal: GI bleeding, GI inflammation, rectal disorder, abnormal hepatobiliary function, reflux, dysphagia and amylase increase[21].

F. Genitourinary: polyuria, dysuria, haematuria and urinary tract infection [21,24,29].

G. Nervous system : anxiety, change in the appetite, depression, drowsiness, dizziness, thirst, impotence, loss of libido, sweating, neuropathy and confusion[24,28].

H. Musculoskeletal : arthralgia, myalgia, muscle cramps, stiffness and back pain [30].

I. Blood and Coagulation : Anemia, abnormal differential count, thrombocytopenia, purpura and increase ESR[31].

Over dose and toxicity

Toxic dose of misoprostol have not been determined, however cumulative dose of up to 2200 microgram administered over a period of 12 hours have been tolerated by pregnant women with no serious adverse effect. A dose of 6000 microgram of misoprostol taken orally to induce an abortion resulted in hyperthermia, rhabdomyolysis, hypoxemia, complex acid- base disorder[17].

Following acute misoprostol over dose, sedation, tremor, seizure, dyspnea, abdominal pain, diarrhea, fever, palpitation, hypotension and bradycardia may occur[24]. These symptoms should be treated with supportive therapy. It appears that dialysis would not be useful in promoting the elimination of drug since it is metabolized as fatty acid[24].

Contraindication and warning

Cytotec is contraindicated because of its abortificient property, in women who are pregnant and the women should be advised not to become pregnant while taking cytotec for peptic ulcer. If a woman becomes pregnant while taking it, the use of product should discontinued[24].

Because it is not known whether misoprostol acid is distributed into milk, the manufacturer recommends that misoprostol not tobe used in nursing women since breast-fed infants could develop clinically important diarrhea if the free acid did distribute to the milk[24,28].

Other contraindications:

Misoprostol should not be used in women with the following conditions

1. glaucoma.
2. sickle cell anemia.
3. mitral valve stenosis.
4. uncontrolled seizure.
5. allergy to Misoprostol or other PGs.[32]

Indications and usage of cytotec

1. Misoprostol (cytotec) is indicated for prevention of NSAID-induced gastric ulcer in patient at high risk of complication from gastric ulcer ,e.g. the elderly and the patient with concomitant debilitating disease , as well as patient at high risk of developing gastric ulceration[24,28] .

2. In gynecologic and obstetric purposes

a. it is used so frequently and so effectively for ripening the cervix prior to induction of labor among pregnant women[33].

b. misoprostol is recommended for use with either Mifepriston or Methotroxate for early pregnancy termination[34].

c. it can be used for cervical ripening before surgical abortion in the 1st and 2nd trimester of pregnancy[27].

In addition , several Randomized controlled trials show that :
- misoprostol alone can be effective for early abortion . these trials have used different regimens and dosage level making comparison difficult , but a number of studies have shown high success rates[35,36].

-Misoprostol has also been shown to be safe and effective in inducing labor[8,33,37].

-In the 2nd trimester , for use in management of miscarriage , or in the cases of intrauterine fetal demise[4,27].

-Misoprostol may also be used to control postpartum hemorrhage , particularly when other drugs are unavailable[17,29,36] .

Advantages of Misoprostol

Misoprostol has several advantages over other PGs currently used for termination of pregnancy or labor induction these are :

-It is supplied in tablet form [38].

-Does not required refrigeration[38] .

-It is available and cheap[38].

-Has less serious side effects as myocardial infarction or bronchspasm which can be caused by PG E2 and PG F2 alpha[17] .

Teratogenisity of misoprostol

In cases in which misoprostol failed to terminate pregnancy congenital abnormality in the infant have been reported these including scalp or skull defect, cranial nerve palsies and limbs defect such as talipes equinovarous, the increase in the uterine pressure related to the uterine contraction or vascular spasm may be the cause of these teratogenic effects[10]

Mobius syndrome (congenital facial paralysis) and limbs defect have occurred in the infants of women who have taken misoprostol during 1st trimester in an unsuccessful attempt to induce abortion [17].

Routes of administration

1. Oral route.

Misoprostol is designed and licensed for oral use. the oral administration of it is associated with rapid onset of action[14].

It is well absorbed by the oral route , with peak plasma concentration achieved in approximately 30 minute and decline rapidly thereafter[17]. the systemic bioavailability of orally administered misoprostol is one third that vaginal misoprostol [39].

2. Vaginal route.

Vaginal administration of misoprostol result in slower increase and lower peak plasma concentration of misoprostol acid than oral administration but over all exposure to the drug is increase[17].

It has been shown that the effect of misoprostol on reproductive tract is increase and gastrointestinal side effects are decreased if the oral preparation of misoprostol is administered vaginally , when misoprostol tablets are placed in the posterior fornix of the vagina plasma concentration of misoprostol acid peaked in 1-2 hours then decline slowly[17].

3. Sublingual route.

This new route of administration, the misoprostol tablet being very soluble in water was put under the tongue , it was observed that it would dissolve within 10-15 minutes[40] .

This route was chosen because it was consider to be the most vascular area of buccal cavity ,it is also avoid the 1st pass effect through the liver in oral administration and un comfortable vaginal administration[2]

4. Intra cervical route.

Although the result was excellent, the administration of the drug into the cervical canal required skill and instrumentation.

5. Rectal route.

Dosage and dosing interval

Recent studies focus mainly on the optimization of misoprostol dosing regimen by comparing various dosages, dosing interval and route of administration. Various regimens are shown in table (1)[2]

Table (1): induction of 2nd trimester abortion by misoprostol regimen.

references	GA(wks)	Regimens	Mean I-A interval(hrs)
Nuutila et al[41]	12-24	vaginal misoprostol 100 mcg q6h for 36hrs max	23.1
Jain & Mishell[42]	12-22	Vaginal misoprostol 200mcg q12x2	14.5
Herabutya&O-praserawat[43]	15-22	.Vaginal misoprostol 400mcgq12hx2 .Vaginal misoprostol 800mcg q12hx2	33.4 22.3
Jain et al[44]	12-22	.vaginal misoprostol 200mcg q6hX8 .vaginal misoprostol 200mcg q12hx4	13.8 14.0
Wong et al[45]	14-20	.Vaginal misoprostol 400mcg q3hx5 . Vaginal misoprostol 400mcg q6hx3	15.2 19.0
Ho et al[46]	14-21	Mifepristone 200mg+400mcg vaginal misoprostol q3hx5	8.7
Dickinson &Evans[14]	16-21	.Vaginal misoprostol 200mcg q6hx4 . Vaginal misoprostol 400mcg q6hx8	18.2 15.1
Ngai et al[47]	14-20	.mifeprostone 200mg +oral misoprostol 400mcg q3hx5	10.4
Bartley& Baired[48]	12-20	. mifeprostone 200mg +800mcg vaginal misoprostol+oral misoprostol 400mcgq3hx4	6.1
Bebbington et al[49]	12-20	.Oral misoprostol 200mcg q1hx3+oral misoprostol 400mcg q4h	34.5

Successful termination was generally considered to be delivery within 48 hours and ranged from 60 to 100%.

Comparisons between these studies are difficult because of the difference in dosage and dosing interval. The dosage of misoprostol used ranged from 100 to 800 mcg with the dosing intervals every 3-12 hours. In general, low dose misoprostol (100-200 mcg) given at every 6-12 hours results in a longer induction-to-abortion interval [2].

The objectives of this study is to asses and compare the clinical efficacy of oral and vaginal misoprostol in the second trimester pregnancy termination.

Materials and Methods

Study Design and Setting:

This study was conducted as prospective Randomized trial at the department of Obestetric and Gynecology in Baghdad teaching hospital throughout the period between (October 2004- October 2005).

Inclusion criteria:

This study involves (100) pregnant women in their 2nd trimester pregnancy (gestational age between 14-28 weeks) with clear indication for termination of pregnancy, in this study those indications were:

• Missed miscarriage.
• Intrauterine fetal death.
• Fetal congenital anomaly.
• Medical maternal indication.

Exclusion criteria:

• Known hypersensitivity to prostaglandin
• Patient with severe bleeding and sepsis
• Patient with history of Asthma
• Patient with Two or more previous uterine scars
• Patient with severe liver and renal impairment

All patient in this study were recruited from outpatient clinic and admitted to the department of obstetric and gynecology where detailed history and full medical and obstetrical examination was carried out.

The demographic characteristic of each patient were assessed including age, body weight, gravidity, parity, history of previous abortion, previous medical disorder, and gestational age that was determined by last menstrual period and ultrasound examination.

List of investigations were conducted for each patient including complete blood picture, renal function test, liver function, blood group and Rh, serum fibrinogen(in cases of missed abortion and IUD) and ultrasound examination was done for each patient to confirm the diagnosis.

Before introducing in this study, an informed consent was obtained from each patient. In patient with fetal congenital anomalies, the decision of pregnancy termination was taken after proper counseling with both parents regarding compatibility with life and any risk if pregnancy continued. In patient with maternal indication of termination, decision was shared between obstetrician and physician.

The patients were randomized in two groups (50 patients for each):

First group was arranged to receive oral protocol of Misoprostol (cytotec) which consist of oral tablet of 200 microgram every one hour for 3 hours then 400 microgram every 4 hours.

Second group was arranged to receive vaginal protocol, which consist of 400 microgram (2 tablets) vaginally every 4 hours .the misoprostol tablets were placed in the posterior fornix of the vagina with the patient in dorsal position using Sims speculum with few drops of water as lubricant, the tablets not pre-moistened at the time of insertion. At the time of placement of subsequent doses, any remaining undissolved tablets were removed before next tablets were inserted. In both groups, the maximum number of doses was five doses in 24 hours.

All patients were followed in the ward every four hrs with observation of pulse rate, blood pressure, temperature and any systemic symptoms were recorded.

Before next dose given uterine contractions and cervical status were assessed by vaginal examination, if abortion or delivery is imminent there is no need for further doses.

During the period of observation, no additional therapy given unless indicated as analgesia for abdominal pain in form of paracetamol tablet or opiods injection.

When delivery or abortion started no additional oxytocic agents as oxytocin or even ergometrin post abortion or delivery were used.

The induction considered to be started when the patient received the first dose of misoprostol and delivery defined as the time when the fetus was expelled although in some cases placenta delivered at the same time.

If the patient undelivered after 24 hrs of treatment further courses of misoprostol was given in the second 24 hrs unless patient request surgical evacuation e.g. in cases of heavy vaginal bleeding.

In this study, failure of induction is considered if the patient not delivered within 48 hrs.

All patients then followed for 24 hrs post abortion or delivery to monitor immediate post abortion complication with monitoring of vital signs, any systemic symptoms, and vaginal bleeding or any passage of tissue per vaginum.

Ultrasonographic examination was performed to detect any retained product of conception, those women with an empty uterus after misoprostol treatment were discharged, those who still had significant parts of product of conception with vaginal bleeding had an evacuation of retained product and then discharged.

Before discharge, each patient was counseled to report any abdominal pain or discomfort, vaginal discharge, fever, general malaise and passage of any tissue mass vaginally, if any of these symptoms occurred, they asked to return to hospital immediately.

The primary outcome measure of interest in this study was induction to delivery interval measured in hrs. The secondary outcome measure was maternal side effect from medication, need for additional intervention and failure to achieve medical termination of pregnancy.

Statistical analysis:

Descriptive analysis was used to show the mean and standard deviation for age, weight, parity, abortion, induction-delivery interval, number of doses required and total dose of drug used.

Percentage and counts used to described the number of patient responding to treatment or not and who developed side effects.

t-test was used to asses the difference between two means of the variables.

Z-test (test of proportion) was used to asses the difference between variables described by percentage and count.

p-value of less than 0.05 was considered statistically significant.

Results

Description of study groups

A total of 100 women in their 2nd trimester pregnancy were randomized between October 2004 and October 2005. Fifty patients were allocated to the vaginal protocol and fifty women to the oral protocol.

The data from those patients were collected and were included in the group to which the patient was randomized. The groups were comparable with regard to maternal age, body weight, parity, number of previous abortions. The mean gestational age according to last menstrual period and according to the early U/S assessment in the oral group were (22.32 ± 4.08 wks, 20.68 ± 3.72 wks respectively) compared with (21.24 ± 4.56 wks and 19.92 ± 3.77 wks respectively) for vaginal group with no statistical significant difference between them ($p=0.21$ and 0.31 respectively) (table (2)).

We did not exclude women from the trial on the bases of previous one caesarean section. In the oral group 5 patients (10%) had previous cesarean section compared with 6 patients (12%) in the vaginal group, ($p=1$ which is not statistically significant).

24 patients in the orally treated group were primigravida and 26 patients (52%) were multigravida compared with 22(44%) primigravida and 24 (48%) multigravida in the vaginal group with no statistical significant difference between two study groups.

Table (2): Characteristics of patients in both study groups

Variables	Oral group n= 50	Vaginal group n=50	P- value
Age (years)*	27.1 ± 5.49	26.5 ± 6.34	0.614
Weight (Kg)*	70 ± 7.19	71.24 ± 7.38	0.396
Gestational age (wks)* by LMP	22.32 ± 4.08	21.24 ± 4.56	0.214
Gestational age (wks)* By U/S	20.68 ± 3.72	19.92 ± 3.77	0.312
Primigravida (n. and %)	24 (48%)	22 (44%)	0.840
Multigravida (n. and %)	26 (52%)	28 (56%)	0.840
Parity*	2.73 ± 1.11	2.39 ± 1.28	0.159
Abortion*	1.19 ± 1.26	1 ± 1.15	0.432
Previous one C/S	5 (10%)	6 (12%)	1.000

*Result are expressed as mean ± SD
P value < 0.05 is of statistical significance.

Regarding the indication for TOP table (3) shows no statistical significant difference between the treatment groups. In the oral group the indications was missed miscarriage in 21 patient, IUD in19 patients and fetal congenital anomalies in 9 patients versus 20, 7, 12 patients respectively in the vaginal group. Maternal indication was one in each group that patient in the oral group was 40 years old had CNS involvement by metastatic tumor, she was in her 20th weeks of gestation with viable fetus. In the vaginal group the patient was 20 years old in her 19th week of gestation with viable fetus and she had Leukemia on chemotherapy.

Table (3): Indications for termination of pregnancies in both study groups.

Indication	Oral group n.	%	Vaginal group n.	%	P-value
Missed miscarriage	21	42	20	40	1.000
Intrauterine fetal death	19	38	17	34	0.834
Congenital anomalies	9	18	12	24	0.623
Maternal indication	1	2	1	2	0.475
Total	50	100	50	100	

The outcome of therapeutic trial

It has been found in this trial that the successful TOP which means complete uterine evacuation without intervention achieved in 90% of both treatment groups while TOP with surgical intervention occur in 6% (3 patient) in each study group (table 4).

Failure of termination occurs in 4% (2 patients) in the oral group who received course of misoprostol for 48 hours with no response, termination then done by oxytocin infusion in one patient and by dilatation and curettage in the other, while in the vaginal group failure of TOP occur in one patient only who had previous uterine scar and had TOP for IUD, this patient failed to respond after receiving course of treatment for 48 hours, successful TOP achieved by oxytocin infusion.

Discontinuation of treatment occurred in one patient in the vaginal group because of development of allergic reaction to misoprostol which occurred after administration of the 1stdose. The patient then switched to oxytocin infusion for TOP, table (4).

Table (4): the outcome of therapeutic trial in both study groups

Parameters	Oral group N=	%	Vaginal group N=	%	p-value
Successful TOP	45	9	45	90	NS*
TOP with surgical intervention	3	6	3	6	NS*
Failure of TOP	2	4	1	2	NS*
Discontinuation of treatment	0	0	1	2	NS
Total	50	100	50	50	NS*

No significant difference

Induction –Delivery interval

As shown in table (5) the mean induction to delivery interval was significantly shorter for group receiving misoprostol according to the vaginal protocol.

The mean ±(SD) induction to delivery for vaginal group was 10.14± 5.28 hours, whereas that for the oral group was 13.47± 8.93 hours (p =0.028) which is statistically significant.

It has also seen that more patients in the vaginal group were delivered in 24 hours compared with the oral group (95.8% vs 87.5%, p=0.270) which is not statistically significant.

Within the vaginal group 72.9% of women delivered in less than 12 hours compared with 60.4% of women in the oral group (p= 0.270)which is of no significant difference while 27% of the oral group delivered between 12-24 hours compared with 22.9% of the vaginal group (p= 0.819).

Also we found that more women receiving oral misoprostol required more than 24 hrs to achieve successful TOP (12.5% vs 4.1% of vaginal group, p=0.261). For them 2nd course of same protocol given in the second 24 hrs without changing the route of administration or the dose given, table (5).

Table (5): the difference in induction to delivery interval between two study groups

parameters	Oral group N=48	Vaginal group N=48	p-value
Induction to delivery interval (hrs)	13.47 ± 8.93	10.14 ± 5.28	0.028
Delivery in 24 hrs	42 (87.5%)	46 (95.8%)	0.270
Delivery in<12 hrs	29 (60.4%)	35 (72.9%)	0.279
Delivery in 12-24 hrs	13 (27%)	11 (22.9%)	0.819
Delivery in >24 hrs	6 (12.5%)	2 (4.1%)	0.261

*Result expressed as mean ±SD
P value < 0.05 is of statistical significance
Number of patients here is 48 after exclusion of failure and discontinuation of treatment.

Table (6) shows that the mean induction to delivery interval was shorter for groups receiving vaginal misoprostol for both missed miscarriage (7.7 ± 2.5 vs 10.97 ± 7.17 hrs for oral group, p=0.06) and IUD (10.81 ± 3.7 vs 17.36 ± 11.22 hrs for oral group, p=0.14), while for congenital anomalies the mean induction to delivery interval was slightly longer in vaginal group than in the oral group (13.33 ± 8.16 hrs vs 12.62 ± 4.47 hrs respectively, p=0.81).

Table (6): comparison of induction to delivery interval (in hrs) according to indication of pregnancy termination in both study groups

Indication	Oral group	Vaginal group	p-value
Missed miscarriage	10.97 ± 7.17	7.7 ± 2.57	0.06
Intrauterine fetal death	17.36 ± 11.22	10.81 ± 3.7	0.14
Congenital anomalies	12.62 ± 4.47	13.33 ± 8.16	0.81

P value < 0.05 is of statistical significance

Predicting a successful outcome of therapeutic trial deciding the number of doses

Regarding the number of doses of misoprostol required for TOP we found that vaginal group required significantly less number of doses than that required for orally treated group (2.70 ± 1.16 dose vs 4.66 ± 1.27, p= 0.00005) this may be related to the protocol used where the oral protocol use the 1st three doses at interval less than that for vaginal group (table 6).It has been found that more dose of drug required for orally treated group than for vaginal group (1266.6 ± 510.8 mcg vs 1083.3 ± 466.6 mcg respectively, p=0.06) which is not statistically significant. Table (7)

Table (7): comparison of number and total dose of misoprostol in both treatment groups

Parameter	Oral group	Vaginal group	p-value
Number of doses required *	4.66 ± 1.27	2.70 ± 1.16	0.00005
Total dose of drug in mcg	1266.6±510.8	1083.3±466.6	0.063

*Results are expressed as mean ± SD
P value <0.05 is of statistical significance.

As shown in table (8), it was observed that no patient in the oral group achieved successful TOP after one and two doses of misoprostol compared with 4 patients (8.3%),p=0.126 and 22 patients (45.8%) respectively for vaginal group, p=0.0000005 which is statistically significant.

22.9% of vaginally treated women required three doses of misoprostol to achieve successful TOP compared with 18.7% of oral group, p=0.803.

More patients in the oral group required four and five doses of drug for TOP (33.3% and 22.9% respectively) compared with (16.6% and 2.08% respectively for vaginal group)with p=0.097 and 0.005 respectively, the latter was statistically significant.

More than five doses required for 25% of orally treated group compared with 4.1% of vaginally treated women, p=0.008 which is statistically significant.

Table (8): A comparison of response rate at the end of each dose interval between oral and vaginal groups.

Doses	Oral group		Vaginal group		P-value	P value
	n=	%	n=	%		
1 Dose	0	0	4	8.3	0.126	<0.05 is of statistical significance.
2 Doses	0	0	22	45.8	0.0000005	
3 Doses	9	18.75	11	22.9	0.803	
4 Dose	16	33.3	8	16.6	0.097	
5 Doses	11	22.9	1	2.08	0.005	
> 5 Doses	12	25	2	4.1	0.008	

Complications during the trial

Table (9) shows that there were no statistical significant differences in complications between two study groups.

We found that postpartum hemorrhage (blood loss > 500 cc) due to uterine inertia occur in one patient in each group (2% for both group, p=0.475). Blood transfusion was required also for one patient in each group

Surgical intervention under general anesthesia for incomplete abortion required in three patient in each group (6%, p=1). The reason for this intervention in the vaginal group was retained placenta for more than one hour.whereas in the oral group two patient had retained placenta and one patient had retained part of products of conception and developed vaginal bleeding in the 2nd day of abortion, U/S was performed and revealed retained part of product of conception and completion of evacuation done surgically under GA.

Allergic reaction observed in one patient of vaginal group(2%) when the patient after administration of the 1st dose of misoprostol developed urticaria and mild shortness of breath, immediate removal of the tablets from the vagina done and administration of antihistamine and hydrocortisone intravenously then the patient switched to oxytocin infusion for termination of her pregnancy.

No known cases of uterine rupture occur in either group.

Table (9): Intrapartum complications in both study groups

Parameter	Oral group		Vaginal group		P-value
	N	%	N	%	
Post partum hemorrhage > 500 cc	1	2	1	2	0.475
Blood transfusion	1	2	1	2	0.475
Retained placenta for > 1hr	2	4	3	6	1.000
Retained part of product of conception	1	2	0	0	1.000
Ruptured uterus	0	0	0	0	1.000
Allergic reaction	0	0	1	2	1.000

P value <0.05 is of statistical significance.

Side effects of misoprostol

With regard to the side effects after misoprostol administration women treated orally reported significantly more gastrointestinal adverse effects than vaginally treated women (17 (34%) vs. 1(2%), p=0.000009).table (10)
These side effects include nausea which observed in five patient (10%) of oral group compared with only one (2%) in the vaginal group, p=0.206.
Vomiting reported in seven (14%) of oral group compared with no such effect in the vaginal group, p=0.018.

Diarrhea observed in five patients (10%) of oral group compared with no such effect in the vaginal group.

Other reported side effects show no statistical difference between two groups as abdominal pain requiring analgesia in form of oral paracetamol or intravenous opiods which observed in 6% of oral group versus 4% of vaginal group , p=1.

Pyrexia (temperature equal and more than 38 c) reported in three patient (6%) of orally treated group and in four patients (8%) of vaginal group, p=1, this fever resolved spontaneously within 24 hours.

Chills occur in 6% of oral group and 4% of vaginal group, p=1.

Headache also observed in 4% of oral group versus 6% of vaginal group, p=1. Table (10).

Table (10): frequency of each side effect between two study groups

P value of <0.05 is of statistical significant.

Reported side effect	Oral group N	%	Vaginal group N	%	p-value
Gastrointestinal					
Nausea	5	10	1	2	0.205
Vomiting	7	14	0	0	0.018
Diarrhea	5	10	0	0	0.06
Total	17	34	1	2	0.00009
Abdominal pain	3	6	2	4	1.000
Pyrexia(temp>38 C)	3	6	4	8	1.000
Chills	3	6	2	4	1.000
Headache	2	4	3	6	1.000

Differences between the response of Primigravida and multigravida in each study group

1. Oral group

In this group as shown in table (11) we found that the mean± (SD) of induction to delivery interval was significantly shorter in multigravida compared with Primigravida (11.46 ± 8.2 hrs vs. 15.86 ± 9.3 respectively, p=0.013.

It was also observed that more women in multigravida group achieved successful TOP within 24 hours than Primigravida (92.3% vs. 75%

respectively, p=0.038) and 16.6% of Primigravida required more than 24 hours for TOP compared with 7.69% of multigravida, p=0.290.

Regarding the number of doses we found that the mean± (SD) of number of doses was less in multigravida (4.25 ± 1.1 vs. 5.13 ± 1.2 for Primigravida, p=0.0005) table (10).

The same table shows that the total dose of misoprostol in multigravida was significantly less than that needed by Primigravida (1049 ± 537.7 mcg vs. 1454.54 ± 569.6 respectively, p=0.0004).

Table (11): comparison between the response of Primigravida and multigravida in oral group

parameter	Oral group		p-value
	Primigravida.	Multigravida.	
I-D interval in hrs*	15.86 ± 9.34	11.46 ± 8.2	0.01
Delivery in 24 hrs	18 (75%)	24 (92.3%)	0.03
Delivery in >24 hrs	4 (16.6%)	2 (7.69%)	0.29
No. of doses required*	5.13 ± 1.28	4.26 ± 1.15	0.0005
Total dose in mcg*	1454.54 ± 569.65	1049 ± 537.74	0.0004

*Results are expressed as mean ± (SD)
P value <0.05 is of statistical significance.

2. Vaginal group

For this group table (12) shows that the mean (SD) 0f induction to delivery interval was significantly shorter in multigravida than Primigravida (8.09 ± 2.3 hrs vs. 12.56 ± 6.6, p=0.00002).

Within 24 hrs it was observed that no statistical significant difference in number of women who achieved successful TOP (92.8 % of multigravida and 90.9% of Primigravida, p=0.985) and no multigravida took more than 24 hrs compared with two women (9.09%) of Primigravida, p=0.088) which is not statistically significant table (12).

As in the oral group multigravida required less number of doses of misoprostol than primigravida (2.23 ± 0.5 vs. 3.27 ± 1.4 respectively, p=0.00006). Table (11)

Regarding the total dose of misoprostol needed again as in the orally treated women multigravida required less dose than Primigravida (892.3 ± 234.8 mcg vs. 1309.09 ± 646.5 mcg respectively, p=0.00004).table (12).

Table (12): comparison between the response of Primigravida and multigravida in the vaginal group

Parameter	Vaginal group		p-value
	Primigravida	Multigravida	
I-D interval in hrs*	12.56 ± 6.68	8.09 ± 2.34	0.00002
Delivery in 24 hrs	20 (90%)	26 (92.8)	0.985
Delivery in > 24 hrs	2 (9.09%)	0	0.088
No. of doses required*	3.27 ± 1.42	2.23 ± 0.58	0.000006
Total dose in mcg*	1309.09 ± 646.53	892.30 ± 234.8	0.00004

Results are expressed as mean ± SD, p value <0.05 is of significance.

Discussion

The development of safe and effective technique for 2nd trimester abortion and intrauterine fetal death become a major clinical challenge, various methods, including Dilatation and evacuation, oxytocin infusion and amnioinfusion of hypertonic saline or urea, were previously used for 2nd trimester abortion and IUD. Different management protocols are continuously revised to achieve improved success rates and reduced discomfort for the patients. The introduction of PGs in the early 1970s has revolutionized the management protocols in this area. PG analogue alone or in combination with mifeprostone have been shown to be effective for the 2nd trimester abortion and IUD [4].

Karim et al [26] 1989 were the 1st to report on the successful use of PG in the management of IUD, following this the use of PG for management of missed miscarriage and IUD has been extensively researched in many trials where different types of PGs, both natural and synthetic had been used.

In our study we use misoprostol which is a synthetic PG E1 analogue marketed for use in prevention and treatment of peptic ulcer disease, it is in expensive and can be stored at room temperature. Although not registered for such use, misoprostol has been widely used in obstetric and gynecology for cervical priming, medical abortion and induction of labor [2] and compare its efficacy when used orally and vaginally in termination of 2nd trimester pregnancy.

The results of this study are encouraging suggesting that misoprostol alone is an effective agent for TOP whether used orally or vaginally where we achieved success rate of 90% in both routes.

Regarding the efficacy we found that vaginal administration is more effective than oral administration (had shorter induction-to-delivery interval and fewer side effects

It has been found that the efficacy of misoprostol regimen improved when a higher dose (400-800 mcg) is given at a shorter interval (3-4 hours) [2] and that is what was used in our study for the vaginal route.

In the oral protocol we gave 200 mcg (one tablet) every one hour for three hours followed by 400mcg (2 tablets) every four hours. The more frequent oral dosing in the 1st three hrs used to try to increase the serum level beyond that seen with more prolonged dosing interval.

A similar aggressive type of oral dosing has been reported previously to be effective at achieving successful TOP. [50]

Neto et al used 400 mcg of oral misoprostol every 4 hrs with high therapeutic effectiveness and low side effects [49].

This study evaluates the effectiveness of oral and vaginal misoprostol for 2nd trimester termination of pregnancy.

We can divide the result of our study into

1. Complete success: when the patient had complete uterine evacuation without surgical intervention. This was achieved in 90% of both groups.
2. Incomplete success: when the patient had incomplete abortion (retained placenta or parts of products of conception) with surgical intervention. This observed in 6% of both groups.
3. Discontinuation of treatment: this occurred in one patient in the vaginal group who developed allergic reaction to misoprostol.

4. Failure of treatment: when the patient failed to abort or deliver after 48 hrs course of misoprostol, this observed in one patient of vaginal group and two patients of oral group.

Although it has been found that oral misoprostol is as effective as vaginal in the 2nd trimester termination of pregnancy where the success rate is 90% in both groups, this study reveals that vaginally administered misoprostol is superior to orally administered misoprostol in term of induction to delivery or abortion interval, delivery or abortion within 24 hours and number of doses required to achieve successful TOP, tables (4, 5, 7).

Bebbington et al [49] compared two protocols for the use of misoprostol in midtrimester pregnancy termination, taking 114 women in the 2nd trimester of pregnancy and randomized into two groups, group 1 assigned to receive oral misoprostol and group 2 assigned to receive vaginal protocol which is exactly similar to our study. They found that the mean induction to delivery interval was significantly shorter for the vaginal group (19.6 ± 17.5 hrs vs 34.5 ± 28.2 hrs, $p<0.01$) this is longer than what obtained in our study (10.14 ± 5.2 hrs for vaginal group and 13.47 ± 8.9 hrs for oral group, $p=0.028$), also they found that significantly more patients in the vaginal group were delivered within 24 hrs (85.1% vs 39.5%, $p<0.01$) this is in agreement with our study although it not reach statistical significant level(95.8% for vaginal and 87.5% for oral group=0.270).

Dickinson et al [14] compare the efficacy of oral and vaginal misoprostol in 2nd trimester pregnancy termination for fetal abnormality using 84 women with GA of 14-26 weeks and had TOP for fetal abnormality, those women randomized into three groups:

Group 1 (28 patients) received 400 mcg vaginal misoprostol at 6 hrs interval.
Group 2 (29 patients) received 400 mcg oral misoprostol at 3 hrs interval.

Group 3 (27 patients) received a loading dose of 600 mcg vaginally followed by 200 mcg orally at 3 hrs interval.

They found that there was significant difference in the median time to achieve delivery among the three groups, group 1(vaginal) 14.5 hrs (in our study it is 10.14 hrs) versus group 2(oral) 25.5 hrs versus group 3(combined oral& vaginal) 16.4 hrs. This result is in agreement with our study for the 1st two groups although the regimen used is different.

Within 24 hrs of commencement 85% of women in group 1(95.8% in our study), 44.8% in group 2(87.5% in our study) and 74% in group 3.

Dickinson also conclude that in the 2nd trimester TOP vaginal misoprostol regimen of 400 mcg at 6 hrs interval is 1.9 times more likely to result in delivery within 24 hrs than oral regimen of 400 mcg at 3 hrs interval.

Chittacharoen et al [4] studied the effectiveness of oral and vaginal misoprostol in management and delivery of fetal death. Their study involve 80 pregnant women at 16-41 weeks gestation with IUD and randomized them in two groups to receive either 400 mcg of misoprostol orally every 4 hrs or 200mcg vaginally every 12 hrs. They found that orally administered misoprostol is more effective than vaginal where the induction to delivery interval was significantly shorter (13.95±5.63 hrs vs 18.87±10.38hrs) but it associated with more frequent gastrointestinal side effects. This is not in agreement with our study may be due to the use of different regimen. In our study there was 19 women in the oral group had IUD and 7 women in the vaginal group, the induction to delivery interval for them was (17.36±11.22 hrs vs 10.81±3.7 hrs, p=0.1 which is not reach statistical significant level).table (6)

The observed effect is likely due to improved pharmacokinetics associated with vaginal administration as demonstrated by Zeiman et al[51] who compared the absorptive kinetics of misoprostol with oral or vaginal administration, they found that systemic bioavailability of vaginally administered misoprostol is three times higher than that of orally administered misoprostol when determined by area under the curve AUC 360, with vaginal administration peak plasma levels are reached more slowly and are slightly lower but are sustained for up to four hours, the markedly different AUC are likely the result of pre-systemic gastrointestinal or hepatic metabolism that occur with the oral but not vaginal administration.

So the greater bioavailability of vaginal misoprostol may explain why intravaginal misoprostol has been reported to be more effective than orally administered for medical abortion.

Other possible explanation is what has been observed by Danielsson et al [38] who compared the effect of oral and vaginal administration of misoprostol on the uterine contractility, they found that uterine contractility initially increase and then plateaued one hour after oral administration whereas uterine contractility increased continuously for four hours after vaginal administration and maximum uterine contractility was significantly higher after vaginal administration.

Aronsson et al[52] studied the effect of misoprostol on the uterine contractility following different routes of administration (oral, vaginal and sublingual) they found that the 1st effect observed was an increase in uterine tonus which occur significantly shorter time following oral (7.8 minutes) and sublingual(10.7 min) than after vaginal(19.4 min).

The time to maximum tonus elevation was also significantly shorter (39.5, 47.1-51.7 and 62.2 min) for three groups respectively.

Regular uterine contraction developed in all subjects following sublingual and vaginal but not with oral administration. The increase in uterine activity measured in Montevideo unite was significantly higher after 2 hrs and thereafter for sublingual and vaginal treatment than for oral misoprostol. This may explain the more effectiveness of vaginal misoprostol over the orally administered misoprostol.

Our study shows that the complication arising during the trial are infrequent and had no statistical difference between two groups (table 9) as incomplete abortion which observed in three patients of each group who need surgical evacuation under GA in whom the process of evacuation by curettage performed easily with no much harm to the cervix because it was already soft or ripe due to misoprostol effects

Allergic reaction to misoprostol found in only one patient in the vaginal group which necessating discontinuation of drug.

The cause of failure which observed in two patients in the oral group and one in the vaginal group is unclear and it was found that termination by alternative methods done successfully.

No uterine ruptures were observed in either of the study group, there has been concern about the possibility of an increased risk of uterine rupture with the use of PG for induction of labor at term and with the use of misoprostol specifically[53], although there are case report of uterine rupture with misoprostol in the 2nd trimester, it appears to be less frequent event than with induction at term[54,55], it is possible that because the lower segment has not thinned to the extent seen at term and the cervix does not need to dilate as much to achieve the expulsion of the fetus.

It is unclear whether the use of misoprostol increase the risk of uterine rupture in women with previous cesarean section or whether any drug used in similar situation would have the same effects. The number of patients with previous scar in our study is too small to make definitive conclusion (5patients in the oral group versus 6 patients in the vaginal group), our study exclude women with two or more scars.

The maternal misoprostol side effects showed an increase in the incidence of gastrointestinal side effects in form of nausea, vomiting and diarrhea in the orally treated group (10%, 14% and 10% respectively) compared with only one patient in the vaginal group who complain from nausea, this may be due to systemic effect of misoprostol that stimulate smooth muscle contraction especially gastrointestinal tract also it could be due to more frequent dose of oral misoprostol used initially and the total number of doses is more than that used in the vaginal protocol (4.6 vs 2.7).

Other notable side effect was abdominal pain which observed in few patients (3 in the oral group and 2 in the vaginal group) it has been found that the pain is more severe in the vaginally treated group which required opiods analgesia and this may be due to prolonged or sustained effect of vaginally administered misoprostol.

The rest of side effects are infrequent and minimum in both groups and resolved spontaneously with out treatment as fever, headache and chills, table (10).

Regarding the adverse effects of misoprostol Bebbington[49] found that there was increase in febrile morbidity in the vaginal group(25% vs 6.7% ,p=0.04), this is not the case in our study where we found that fever observed in only 6% of oral group and 8% of vaginal group, p=1 which is not significant.

our study shows that misoprostol like other uterotonic agents is more effective in multiparous than in nulliparous women whether used orally or vaginally (table 11, 12) this may be due to increase the sensitivity of the uterus to uterotonic agents as parity increased so misoprostol should be used carefully in multiparous women and some studies exclude women with parity of five and more [7].

Conclusions

This study demonstrates that:

1. Misoprostol (synthetic PG E1 analogue) alone is very effective agent for 2nd trimester termination of pregnancy whether used orally or vaginally with success rate of 90% in both routes.
2. Oral preparation of misoprostol can be used vaginally, by this way the effect of misoprostol on the reproductive tract increase and gastrointestinal adverse effects are decrease.
3. Vaginal administration of misoprostol is more effective than orally administered in termination of 2nd trimester pregnancy in term of shorter induction to delivery or abortion interval, less doses required and fewer adverse effects, this is likely due to improved pharmacokinetics associated with vaginal administration.
4. Intravaginal misoprostol at a dose of 400 mcg at 4 hour intervals is effective regimen to achieve successful TOP.
5. Adverse effects of misoprostol are minimum and self limiting.
6. Misoprostol whether used orally or vaginally is more effective in multiparous than in nulliparous women so it should be used carefully in grandmultiparous women.

Recommendations

1. Trials needed to optimize the dose and dosage intervals of misoprostol in the 2nd trimester termination of pregnancy.
2. Trials required to find the maximum dose beyond which further administration of misoprostol is of no benefit.
3. Since oral preparations not dissolve completely when used vaginally, development of preparations that dissolve more completely, such as gel or suppositories is recommended.

References

1. Mackenzie IZ. Labor induction including pregnancy termination for fetal anomaly. In James DK, Steer PhJ, Weiner CP, Conik B, (ed). High risk pregnancy (management options), volume 2. London, Harcourt publisher. 1999; 1079-1101.
2. Sak Oi S, Pak Ch. Prostaglandin for induction of second trimester termination and intrauterine death. Best practice and research clinical obstetric and gynecology 2003; 17(5):765-775.
3. Scott RJ, Di Saia JPh, Hammond ChB, Spellacy WN. Danforths obstetric and gynecology, Philadelphia, Lippincott William and Willkins.eighth edition. 1999; 571.
4. Apichart Ch, Yongyoth H, Piyaporn P. A randomized trial of oral and vaginal misoprostol to manage delivery in cases of fetal death. Obstet Gynecol 2003; 101(1):70-73.
5. Second trimester miscarriage. In Stuart Campbell, Christop Lees, Obstetric by Ten-teachers, London, Arnold.17th edition. 2000; 263-271.
6. Mohajer MP. Management of fetal anomalies. In Luesley DM, Baker PhN. (ed). Obstetric and Gynecology (An evidence-based text for MRCOG), London, Harcourt publisher, 1st edition, 2004; 221-224.
7. Makhlouf AM, Al-Hussaini TK, Habib DM, and Makarem MH. Second trimester pregnancy termination, comparison of three different methods. Obstet Gynecol 2003; 23(4): 407-411.

8. Hayman R. Induction of labor. In Luesely DM, Baker PhN. (ed). Obstetric and Gynecology (An evidence-based text for MRCOG), London. Hartcourt publisher, 1st edition. 2004; 327-338.
9. Zikopoulos KA, Papanikolaou EG, Kalantaridou SN, Tsanadis GD, Plachouras NI, Dalkalitsis NA and Paraskevaidis EA. Early pregnancy termination with vaginal misoprostol before and after 42 days gestation. Hum Reprod 2002; 17(12): 3079-3083.
10. Christine S, Matre, Bouchard Ph, and Spitz IM. Medical termination of pregnancy, N Eng J Med 2000; 342(13): 946-950.
11. Kenny L. Contraception, sterilization and termination of pregnancy, In Luesley DM, Baker PhN.(ed) Obstetric and Gynecology (An evidence-based text for MRCOG).London .Harcourt publisher, 1st edition. 2004; 514-523.
12. Grudzinskas JG. Miscarriage, ectopic pregnancy and trophoblastic disease. In Edmond DK. Dewhurts textbook of obstetric and gynecology for postgraduate, London, 6th edition. 1999;61- 74.
13. Inflammation, arthritis and NSAIDs. In Laurence DR, Bennett PN, Brown MJ. Clinical pharmacology, Edinburgh, Churchill Livingston, 8th edition. 1997; 249-266.
14. Dickinson JE, Evan ShF. A comparison of oral misoprostol with vaginal misoprostol administration in 2nd-trimester pregnancy termination of fetal abnormality. Obstet Gynecol 2003; 101, (6):1294-1299.
15. Misoprostol / Cytotec by drdoc on-line (internet work)
16. Bundy G, Lincoln F, Nelson N. Novel PG synthesis. Annual of the New York academy of science 1971; 76-90.

17. Goldberg AB, Greenberg MB, Darney PhD. Misoprostol and pregnancy. N Eng J Med 2001; 344(1):38.
18. Monk JP, Clissold SP. Misoprostol: a preliminary review of its pharmacodynamic and pharmacokinetic properties and therapeutic efficacy in the treatment of peptic ulcer disease, drugs 1987; 33:1-30.
19. Collins PW. Development and therapeutic role of synthetic PG in peptic ulcer disease. J Med Chemist 1986; 29: 437-3.
20. Collins PW, Pappo R, Dajan EZ. Chemistry and synthetic development of misoprostol. Dig Dis Sci 1985; 30: 114-75 (IDIS 208364).
21. Al-Tikreeti R, Muhauder S, The Treatment of Incomplete and Missed Abortion with Oral Misoprostol (accepted for publication in Iraqi postgraduate medical journal 2005; 4(4).
22. Induction of labor by Oral and vaginal misoprostol, (internet-work).
23. Sherman DJ, Frenkel E, Pansky M, Caspi E. Bukovsky and Langer R. Balloon cervical ripening with extra-amniotic infusion saline or PG E2. A double blind Randomized controlled study. Obstet Gynecol 2001; 97(3): 375.
24. Cytotec (misoprostol) prescribing information dated 1991 Aug 12. In: Physician's desk reference, 47th edition. Motval, NJ: Medical Economics Inc. 1993; 2251-3.
25. Nicholson PA. A review of the therapeutic efficacy of misoprostol, a prostaglandin E1 analogue. South Africa medical Journal. 1988; 74: 56-8 (IDIS 2493363).
26. Karim A. Antiulcer PG misoprostol: single and multiple dose pharmacokinetic profile, Prostaglandins 1989; 33 (suppl): 40-50.

27. Simmonds K, Yanow S, Misoprostol for self induced abortion sharing responsibility, women society and abortion world wide. New York: Alan Guttmacher Institute 1999.
28. Searle.Cytotec (misoprostol) product information from the American Hospital formulary service. Skokie, IL; 1988 dec.
29. El-Refaey H, O Brien P, Morafa W. Use of misoprostol in prevention of postpartum hemorrhage, Br J Obstet Gynecol 1997; 104: 336-339.
30. Jiranek GC, Kmmy MB, Sounders DR. Misoprostol reduces gastrointestinal injury from one week of Aspirin an endoscopic study. Gastroenterology 1989; 96:656-61 (IDIS 250825).
31. Herting RL, Nissen CH. Overview of misoprostol clinical experience. Dig Dis Sci. 1986; 31 (suppl): 47-54.
32. short cut to misoprostol in obstetric and gynecology. Summary of evidence.
33. Senior J, Marshall K, Sangha R, Clayton JK. Invitro characterization of prostanoid receptor on human myometerium at term pregnancy. Br J Pharma 1993; 108: 501-506.
34. Creinine, Vitti nghoff E, Methotroxate and misoprostol versus misoprostol alone for early abortion. A randomized controlled trial, J A M A 1994; 272 (15): 1190-5.
35. Jone ETM, Makin JD, Manfeldt. Randomized trial of medical evacuation and surgical curettage for incomplete miscarriage. Br J Med 1995; 311:662.
36. Chung H, Lee S, Cheung L. Spontaneous abortion: A randomized controlled trial comparing surgical evacuation with conservative management using misoprostol. Fertility and Sterility 1999; 71(6): 1054-1059.

37. Tong OS, Wong KS, Jang LC. Pilot study on the use of repeated doses of misoprostol in termination of pregnancy at less than 9 weeks of gestation. Adv. Contracept 1999; 15(3): 211-6.
38. Danielson KG, Marious L, Rodriguez A, Wong PYK, and Bygedman M. Comparison between oral and vaginal administration of misoprostol on uterine contractility. Obstet Gynecol 1999; 93(2): 275.
39. Corten SJ, Bouldin Sh, Blust D, and O Brien WF. Safety and efficacy of misoprostol orally and vaginally. A randomized trial. Obstet Gynecol 2001; 98(1): 107.
40. Oi Shan Tang, Schweer H, Seyberth HW, Sharon WH, and Pak Chung Ho. Pharmacokinetics of different route of administration of misoprostol. Hum Reprod 2002; 17(2): 332-336.
41. Nuutila M, Toivonen, Ylikorkala O and Halmesmaki E. A comparison between two doses of intravaginal misoprostol and gemeprost for induction of second trimester abortion. Obstet Gynecol 1997; 90: 896-900.
42. Jain JK and Mishell DR. A comparison of intravaginal misoprostol with prostaglandin E2 for termination of second trimester pregnancy. N Eng J Med 1994; 5:290-293.
43. Herabutya Y and O-Prasertsawat P. second trimester abortion using intravaginal misoprostol. Int J Gynecol Obstet 1998; 60:161-165.
44. Jain JK, Kuo J and Mishell R. A comparison of two dosing regimens of intravaginal misoprostol for second trimester pregnancy termination. Obstet Gynecol 1999; 93:571-575.
45. Wong KS, Ngai CSW, Yeo ELK. A comparison of two regimens of intravaginal misoprostol for termination of second trimester

pregnancy: a randomized comparative trial. Hum Reprod 2000; 15:709-712.
46. Ho PC, Chan YF and Lau W. Misoprostol is as effective as gemeprost in termination of second trimester pregnancy when combined with mifepristone: A randomized comparative trial. Contraception 1996; 53:281-183.
47. Ngai SW, Tang OS and Ho PC. Randomized comparison of vaginal (200 mcg every 3h) and oral (400 mcg every 3h) misoprostol when combined with mifepristone in termination of second trimester pregnancy. Hum Reprod 2000; 15:2205-2208.
48. Bradly J and Baired DT .A randomized study of misoprostol and gemeprost in combination with mifepristone for induction of abortion in second trimester pregnancy. Obstet Gynecol 2003; 109:1290-1294.
49. Bebbington MW, Kent N, Lim k and Gagnon A.A randomized controlled trial comparing two protocols for the use of misoprostol in midtrimester pregnancy termination. Am J Obstet Gynecol 2002; 187:853-857.
50. Batioglu S ,Tonguc E, Haberal A, Celikk anat H, Bagis T. Midtrimester termination of complicated pregnancy with oral misoprostol. Adv. Contracept 1997; 13:55-61.
51. Zieman M, Frong SK, Benowitz NL, Banskter D and Darney. Absorption kinetics of misoprostol with oral or vaginal administration .Obstetrics Gynecol 1997; 90(1): 88-91.
52. Aronsson A, Bygdman M, Danielsson G. Effect of misoprostol on uterine contractility following different routes of administration. Hum Reprod 2004; 19(1):81-84.

53. Hill DA, Chez RA, Quinlon J, Fuentes A, La Combe J. Uterine rupture and dehiscence associated with intravaginal misoprostol cervical ripening. J Reprod. Med. 2000; 45:823-6.
54. Chen M, Shih JC, Chiu WT, Hsich FJ. Separation of cesarean scar during second trimester intravaginal misoprostol abortion. Obstet Gynecol 1999; 94:840.
55. Berghahn L, Christenson D, Droste S. Uterine rupture during second trimester abortion associated with misoprostol. Obstet Gynecol 2001; 98:976-7.

MoreBooks! publishing

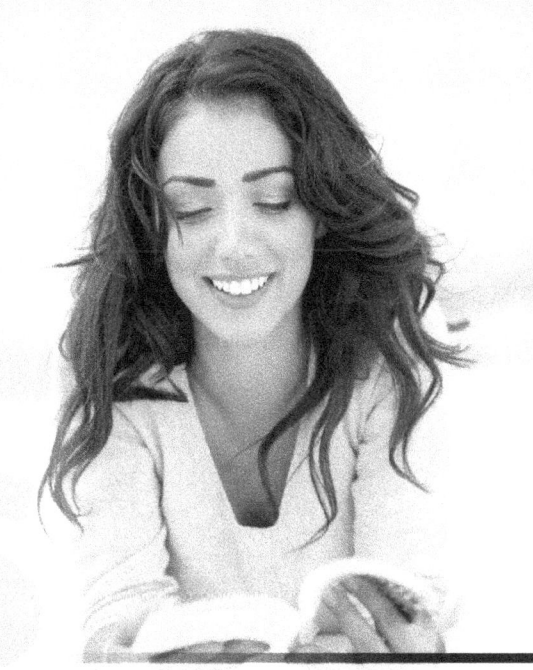

i want morebooks!

Buy your books fast and straightforward online - at one of world's fastest growing online book stores! Environmentally sound due to Print-on-Demand technologies.

Buy your books online at
www.get-morebooks.com

Kaufen Sie Ihre Bücher schnell und unkompliziert online – auf einer der am schnellsten wachsenden Buchhandelsplattformen weltweit! Dank Print-On-Demand umwelt- und ressourcenschonend produziert.

Bücher schneller online kaufen
www.morebooks.de

VDM Verlagsservicegesellschaft mbH
Heinrich-Böcking-Str. 6-8
D - 66121 Saarbrücken
Telefon: +49 681 3720 174
Telefax: +49 681 3720 1749
info@vdm-vsg.de
www.vdm-vsg.de